A GUIDE IN PLAIN ENGLISH:

K.I.S.S.

(KEEP IT SIMPLE STEPS TO)

BIRTH PREPARATION

This book delivers birth to you in a gentle, relaxed and empowering way. The most essential birthing basics in a perfectly compact bundle

CLARE CURTIS

BE EMPOWERED. INFORM YOURSELF ABOUT BIRTH - A GUIDE IN PLAIN ENGLISH

CLARE CURTIS

All information is correct at the time of publishing to the best of the authors knowledge. The author takes no responsibility for the action you take as a result of this book. This book is not medical advice. The author is a mother of two children with an interest in women's health and global issues our world faces. Knowledge is power. Be empowered!

Essex, UK

K.I.S.S.
(KEEP IT SIMPLE STEPS TO)
BIRTH
PREPARATION

Clare Curtis

CONTENTS

PROLOGUE

Having had a first birth experience that was anything but empowering and positive - I retrained to specialise in women's pre and post natal care and went on to have a second birth experience at home that was one of the most empowering and beautiful experiences of my life.

I am driven to support and help as many women as possible have positive pregnancy and birth experiences and I have taught hundreds of women pregnancy yoga and birth preparation classes for over five years.

Sometimes the concept of preparing for birth can be overwhelming, sometimes it's an after thought. This book will help you determine what you need to prioritise.

This is a quick and essential guide for any couple embarking on the birth of a new baby. The emphasis is on all the basic information women and men should be aware of in relation to how a woman's body is perfectly designed and how naturally birth can flow.

It is ideal for busy people and those endeavouring to have as empowered and positive a birth experience as possible.

The guide has tips and tools and I urge you to explore them all in some capacity.

I wish you a healthy, empowered pregnancy, birth and
journey into motherhood.

Much love

Clare
Xx

1.
A POSITIVE BIRTH EXPERIENCE

It should almost go without saying as to why every woman should have a positive birth experience. However, sadly we are bombarded with stories and media portrayals of birth that are incredibly damaging. The thing is we don't know what we don't know.

We were not taught about the absolute perfection of the design of the human body in school. It is the finest machine and has the finest architecture, it is complex however everything has a purpose, it is all by design.

There are no mistakes with our bodies if we learn more about what it is capable of, this guide will help you and your birth partner explore why birth SHOULD be no different than any other bodily function. We need to learn to surrender and let it flow.

If we can learn to trust our bodies and reconnect with our innate wisdom then we can tune in and follow the flow of birth, as nature intended. So thank you for taking the first step, you and your baby will be grateful for the best possible start in life. It can make all the difference to your experience as a parent.

WHY A POSITIVE BIRTH IS IMPORTANT

Firstly all the right hormones will be present throughout birth and when your baby is in your arms. This can help with healing, bonding and milk supply (if you intend to breast feed). If you have low cortisol levels (stress hormones) then this can help you adjust and ease you into parenthood more gently.

When the majority of your birth is positive and you feel in control of the decision making process, it is empowering! You are not a patient and women have been giving birth for generation upon generation, they did not need to visit a hospital but called upon an experienced midwife who could guide them and support them through the process of birth. If you have an empowered mindset, you are realistic and understand what your body is doing the experience can leave you incredibly proud of what you have done.

If you are informed you and your bath partner can ask relevant questions and make the best decisions for you. This will mean you feel safe and heard and making choices and align them with what you are comfortable with.

A positive birth experiences can impact your future in ways you may not yet fathom. You will have a deep respect for what your body is capable of and this will carry you forward in life. Understanding just how miraculous and amazing our bodies are can shift your perspective. In part a positive birth experience will enable you to TRUST yourself and your instincts as you move forward into parenthood

CONVERSLY

Healing can be more lengthy, this includes physically, mentally and emotionally. If you are unprepared and not moving or getting into optimum positions then you may prolong the birth. This will take longer to heal from physically, imagine running two marathons one after the other if you only had to run one!

Your hormones may not flow how they should due to interventions and this can result in milk supply being inhibited and feel good hormones for bonding taking longer to come through.

Birth trauma can occur if you feel unsafe or not heard during your birth experience. A negative birth experience sadly can lead to some women experiencing Post Natal Depression (PND) or Post Natal Anxiety. In some cases a woman or her birth partner can later go on to experience PTSD symptoms, frequently mis-diagnosed as PND.

However long term a negative birth experience may prevent you wishing to have further children in the future.

SO WHAT IS A POSITIVE EMPOWERED BIRTH?

- Feeling you are coming from a place of knowledge and confidence

- Feeling calm and in a position to make the best decisions at the time

- Understanding you have a CHOICE and feeling as though you've made the right choice for you at the time with the information available to you

- Remembering you have rights over your body. You have autonomy over your body, birth and baby.

- Remembering that the people around you are there to assist IF you need it, you are not a patient

- You are a woman who knows her body and what she is capable of, you are in tune with your body and your babies needs and if there is something you need assistance with then it is there for you.

- Knowing that no matter what, you have felt empowered in labour and despite any surprises you have been able to remain calm and use your B.R.A.I.N. (More on this to follow)

- Being happy with the choices you have made in the
  unknown unique situation that is YOUR birth.

- Knowing with certainty you are a powerful, strong,
  smart woman. Yes you are!

2.
MINDSET PREPARATION

Mindset preparation is vital. If you have a positive outlook, if you surround yourself with people that know there is a better way to birth then you will see how tangible a good and healthy experience can be.

We live in a culture where people will often share their a story of birth, the duration, the pain relief, any twists and turns that took place. We see so much imagery on TV and in films portraying birth in a way that seems that a woman is powerless.

If your first exposure to birth was a film or a difficult birth story was in your mind when you next saw a birthing woman giving birth on TV then your perspective of birth is being shaped. Western culture continues to reinforce birth in a negative way in the media and this is imprinted in our neural pathways.

Mindset preparation is rewriting the script so your mind and subsequently your body KNOW the truth about how your body and birth is designed.

"SURRENDER AND ALLOW BIRTH TO FLOW"

However, an empowered woman giving birth in a birthing pool gently does not make good drama, a woman giving birth in her shower at home, or on all fours roaring her baby out does not make good TV. Can you imagine if the truth about birth was mainstream? What a different kind of world we would live in.

People do have negative and difficult, sometimes tragic birth experiences, this is not deniable. However in some difficult birth cases it could have been preventable if the woman and her birth partner had invested time in educating themselves and learning and practicing tools and techniques that will support them. There is no judgement here I was one of those women with my first birth. I can look back with the knowledge I have now and see where it went wrong. This is not to do with the medical system, this is to do with my mindset and preparation, the way in which I was not fully aware of what I was capable of, I did not prioritise ensuring that I had tools to help me.

When I went to a hospital I became a dis-empowered patient the moment there was something happening I didn't understand, I did not ask questions and as a result, interventions where made and I ran two marathons instead of one. During birth and for eighteen months after.

So, cautionary tale aside I invite you to make the birth experience your project, not the nursery decor, or the adorable outfits, what matters most is the experience and start you have on your baby's Birth Day. The most important day of their life, the day they come into the world for the very first time.

So start now, think about what you surround yourself with, the words you use what you allow yourself to listen to when it comes to pregnancy and birth scenarios. Speak to those people that have not shared their positive birth experiences, there are more than you may realise and the numbers are growing. They do not share their stories often because it may come across as gloating and they are sensitive to the women that had a different experience, however they do have awe inspiring stories. Not always perfect, not always pretty however they are real, empowering and inspiring so seek them out.

This is your opportunity to re - learn what you've convinced yourself you already know but may not be true.

FLIP YOUR FEAR

You may need to begin by flipping any fears you may have about a physiological/ vaginal delivery, or even about a medicalised or interventions that take place. All of the fear needs to be rationalised, processed and unlearned.

Here's an exercise to FLIP Birth fear and created a
positive perspective on aspects you're concerned about

- Turn the negative into a positive
- Write it down
- Choose to believe the positive

If there is anything you or your birth partner write it down
and reframe it. For example:

- Fear of lying on a bed - "What it means to me is becoming a patient, being still and not helping my baby." REFRAME - I can use the bed as a prop, I can still be on all fours leaning on the bed, it may be appropriate whilst listening to relaxation tracks

- IV Drip - "I am fearful being induced can make labour more intense and create further interventions." REFRAME - Think of the drip as a tree of life for labour helping to bring my baby into the world, if I remain calm I can still breathe my baby into the world.

- Midwife or caregiver - "An unknown person" - REFRAME - An experienced person present for reassurance and safety that understands labour and birth and has seen it many times before. Note: It is ok to ask for an alternative caregiver or ask the caregiver to communicate in a way that your will respond to positively.

OR

- Fear of Pain - Understanding the process of birthing your baby. It is a natural process and the muscles contracting in the uterus will hurt as this is the only time it is used, it is all temporary. The more you can focus on relaxing, surrendering to what your body needs you to do and focus on your breath the more likely you are to notice a real issue instinctively. Your body will tell you.

It is the only thing that can be painful and will bring a positive outcome.

3.
MIRACLE OF YOU

On the whole humans rarely have a full comprehension of what our bodies are capable of. We still have a lot to learn and we are capable of so much more than we realise.

When it comes to birth we have become immersed in a medical ways of thinking for what is a natural process. Whilst intervention may be required in some instances physiologically it is better for us to recognise women are perfectly designed to grow a human being and to birth a human being!

Women however have lost ancestral knowledge about birth, in some cultures children learn about birth at a young age perhaps watching other women give birth in close knit communities. Women are all fully on board, unquestioning that birth is a natural process. They may take themselves off somewhere they feel safe and they birth through instinct and trust and what they have observed in women before them.

However, we seem to have forgotten.

No other animal is assisted when giving birth. We have the health service which is fantastic to safe guard us and our babies, however we aren't a patient just because we may choose give birth in an hospital.

Look at nature, the intricacy of trees, leaves, flowers, birds.... all designed perfectly. Why would the design of the most advanced species on the planet be anything other than perfect?

Would we really be so flawed that our bodies can not birth the phenomenal miracle we can create inside our wombs? I don't think so.

DID YOU KNOW....?

THE UTERUS

- A woman's uterus can expand up to 500X its normal size! It goes from the size of a pear to that of a water melon! It supports our baby, amniotic fluid and placenta! Just this part of us alone is amazing!

- Despite the uterus expanding to this size once your baby is born it will shrink back to it's normal size again.

THE CERVIX

- Your cervix is a ring of muscle, a sphincter muscle. This muscle ALONE supports and holds the weight of your growing baby, the amniotic fluid and placenta!

- Only when it is near your due date does it begin to soften, only as labour starts and baby is ready does it begin to open.

- Your cervix is directly correlated to your jaw. A relaxed jaw is a relaxed cervix!

MORE INCREDIBLE PERFECT DESIGN.....

THE PLACENTA

- The placenta is an organ your body MAKES when you fall pregnant. You make an actual organ! Phenomenal!

- The placenta chooses what to take, give and store for your baby

- The placenta which looks very much like a tree does a similar job, connecting your baby to life giving nutrients and nourishment whilst also purifying the environment

- In some cultures if a baby is born unresponsive the placenta is massaged and warmed to stimulate the organ and revive the baby*

- After birth if the placenta is eaten or steamed and put into capsules for the mother it can help reduce blood loss, improve healing, enable milk supply to occur more quickly and provide much needed energy and help with hormone balance

(*Source: Placenta the Forgotten Chakra - Robert Lim)

RECAP

In this section you have learnt:

- What a positive and empowered birth is
- Why we need to work on our mindset
- Our capability and incredible human design

Your action to take is:

- Reframe any fear or misconceptions you have about
  birth
- Write them down
- Surround yourself with positive birth stories
- If you have had a negative or traumatic birth prior to
  this pregnancy seek support to detached from any
  negative emotion relating to this

4.
VITAL ROLE OF A BIRTH PARTNER

"TEAMWORK TO MAKE THE DREAM WORK"

Our birth partner needs to know the importance of mindset, the importance and power of words in birth and the impact this may have on a birthing mother. They should also understand the crucial effect the environment has when a woman gives birth. Overall a birth partners role is to ensuring the birthing mother feels safe, protected and loved. The body and mind are intwined during birth and there is a logical, biological reason for this.

To get into the headspace of a birthing mother we need to understand a little about how the brain works.

So here is is... Simplified!

PRIMITIVE BRAIN & NEOCORTEX STIMULATION

We have a part of the brain called the Neocortex, this is
the intellectual part of our brain we use on a daily basis,
helping us to make decisions such as "Is it safe to cross
the road?" "What tasks do I need to complete today?"
"What's the square root of Pi?"

We also have a Primitive or Reptilian part of our brain
which is far more instinctive. This part of our brain is
used in our self preserving behaviours such as our fight
or flight responses, sex and birth.

WHY IS THIS IMPORTANT?

Birth is primitive, it comes from a part of us we don't use
on a daily basis. For example noises sometimes made in
labour can be very animalistic and are completely
natural! Often women won't know where the noises are
coming from and they may never be able to make them
again, they come from a deep unknown place.

If we are unaware that birth is a primal instinct when we
are giving birth we may be fearful of how we feel when
our body takes over. This is why we must surrender to
the birthing process and enable it to flow.

Just like all animals giving birth in a secluded place we
are also designed to birth like this. A place we feel safe

and where we can connect to our primitive brain and get into our "zone" or the instinctive headspace and focus.

Distractions that require us to come out of this primitive headspace or to use our logical neocortex can slow down labour because our rational thinking brain is being used rather than the instinctive primal part of our brain.

If we are fearful in birth, just like any other animal, this can hinder the process until we feel safe again. In the past this may have protected our baby. For example a woman is in a cave giving birth, her partner is ensuring the space remains a safe one for her to give birth in. IF a tiger was to come and explore the cave the woman would no longer be safe to give birth, labour would have to stop so she could run and labour would have to stop. It's basic survival, our fight and flight responses will protect us.

Although there aren't tigers that may be a threat some people can perceive a situation as a threat. For example would a woman feel safe if during birth there was a huge crash outside the room she was birthing in? Or would she become very aware of her surroundings and subconsciously would her body respond in a protective manner until she knows she is safe?

If she did even momentarily feel unsafe what do you think would happen to the flow of labour? When you can comprehend the logic behind this response you may also begin to see why the environment should be conducive to birth. Why a woman must feel safe. Why the care givers should treat her respectfully and listen to her needs. If these basic environmental factors are not in place the biologic response will be to slow labour down or stop altogether. It is the birth partners role to ensure that the mother feels safe and supported at all times.

5.

ENVIRONMENT

SPHINCTERS LAW

Most people haven't heard of this, however it sheds a lot of light on what is wrong with the way we treat birth in modern culture. Sphincters Law can also go some way to explain more fully why birth can slow down, stop and how some environments are not ideal for a woman to birth in.

Sphincters Law was observed by a world wide renowned midwife called Ina May Gaskin. Her work has been instrumental in helping many women give birth and educate many women around the world that support women during pregnancy and birth. A real life hero.

INA MAY DISCOVERIES

"The vagina and the cervix, not just the anus and the urethra are sphincters, circular muscles surrounding the opening of organs which are required to empty themselves at appropriate times.

These openings ordinarily remain closed but have the ability to open as widely as needed when necessary.

Each of the organs are able to contract rhythmically as it fills, until it reaches the point of urgency, then sphincter relaxes so that urination, defecation, or birth, takes place." *

She goes on to say:

- - Your sphincters respond to your environment and are unresponsive to demands

- Relaxation and privacy is important

- Your sphincter muscles (cervix) will contract potentially in response to people coming in and out of the birthing room.

- Often at the arrival to hospital the opening of your cervix may slow down or stop entirely. This is important to remember if you choose to allow a vaginal examination (VE). You may be less dilated when you arrived than if you were relaxed at home for example.

- If you feel threatened in any way your cervix may close completely. Please be aware of this, it emphasises how the environment is important to a

labouring woman. Feeling safe and relaxed will
physically help labour flow and your cervix to dilate.

CONTEXT

Sometimes it's helpful to put context around Sphincters
Law.

I'm going to touch on a couple of things to help you think
about how this law is relevant in YOUR daily life.

- If you are going to the toilet in a public setting, would
  you feel comfortable if there was no door? If anyone
  can walk past and see you. Would you be able to
  relax? Will you feel vulnerable at all? How would your
  experience be? Awkward. Rushed or pressured?

- If someone needs to use the same toilet as you and is
  banging on the door telling you to hurry up, or you
  have to leave to go somewhere and you're running
  late - What does that kind of pressure have on your
  experience?

Our sphincter muscles do not respond well to this kind of
pressure or lack of privacy.

Here are the most important features of sphincters and their function according to several factors:

1. Sphincters open best in conditions of privacy and intimacy
2. Sphincters open best without time limits
3. Sphincters are not under the voluntary control of their owner. They do not obey orders, such as 'urinate now!', 'push!', or 'poop!'
4. Sphincters, however, do respond well to praise, if there happens to be another person in the proximity of the sphincter's owner. This other person might be the birthing partner or a midwife assisting a woman giving birth
5. The opening of sphincters can be facilitated by laughter (the owner's)
6. When a person's sphincter is in the process of opening, it may suddenly close if that person becomes frightened, upset, embarrassed, or self-conscious. This is because high levels of adrenaline in the bloodstream do not encourage the opening of the sphincters
7. The state of relaxation of the mouth and jaw is directly correlated to the ability of the cervix, the vagina, and the anus to open to full capacity. A relaxed and open mouth favours a more open vagina and cervix.

Reference: "Ina May's Guide to Childbirth"

SOUND

In connection to what we have covered so far in relation
to our primitive brain, instincts and Sphincters Law - I
would like you to begin considering sound.

During birth a woman may make lots of sounds
instinctively. Be comfortable making sounds as they will
help your jaw relax, (which as already stated is correlated
with your cervix) and it will help your breath work (more
on that later).

By both you and your partner acknowledging this and
practicing during pregnancy you will be less inhibited
during labour.

Remember any sounds that come from you during labour
come from a deep ancestral knowing. They are
empowering. Screaming as we so often see in the media
is disempowering and not a constructive use of your
energy. Use your energy wisely!

PRACTICE

- Oooooh's & Aaahhhs - Make you feel less inhibited,
  releases tension in your body, abdominally and in
  your jaw. The long breath out calms your central
  nervous system.

- Moo like a cow! - This relaxes the mouth and the jaw, opening up your (sphincters) cervix. Often women use this sound sometimes when on all fours. The gentle pressure of the sound going through your body helps send energy down.

- Om - A sonic massage for your baby in pregnancy and birth. A deep sound which again sends energy inwards.

- Pppffff - Also known as horse lips, Blowing out through the mouth with relaxed lips, releases tension in the mouth and opens the throat, therefore the cervix!

- As we make these sounds you can imagine the breath sending your energy down, a bit like the plunger on a cafetière, slowly pushing downwards. Downwards like your baby through the birthing canal.

EXERCISE:

- Next time you go to the toilet to poo, providing you're not at work or in a public place! I suggest you Moo! on the toilet. You may feel a bit silly however you will see how much easier it is for you to poo. This is a great exercise for both of you to try, it starts to break down inhibitions and proves how effective this knowledge and the breath with sound can be.

- Some women during pregnancy also experience constipation, this is a useful technique to know if needed at any point.

- I've also used this technique with my children!

- Have fun with it ;-)

6.
HOW THE BRAIN WORKS - MORE

BIRTH PARTNER ROLE

Because it is so important and because sometimes the birthing partner may need a little persuasion about how the can be involved and why, this chapter is dedicated to them. If they only read one chapter initially let it be this chapter.

So birth partners! Think back to the cave men days when a man would protect the entrance to the cave, ensuring predators couldn't threaten or maim a woman whilst they gave birth. The woman could give birth feeling safe, knowing it was ok for her to bring her baby into the world. The protection is one role of the birth parter.

- If a woman is not relaxed then her instincts and her body are telling her if she births now when in "danger" or when there is a perceived threat then her baby will be unsafe and she herself may need to flee or fight. YOU NEED TO KEEP HER RELAXED.

- Our primitive brain is protecting us. Therefore it is imperative a birthing woman feels entirely safe and relaxed in her environment and around her caregivers. YOU NEED TO ENSURE SHE FEELS SAFE.

- Whilst we no longer have the threat of a sabre toothed tiger, other threats are intrusive people, unsuitable birth environments and other surprises that may come up as labour unfolds. BE PREPARED, BE CALM.

- The birth partner is required to help set and create the right atmosphere for the mother to birth. ENSURE THE ENVIRONMENT IS RIGHT FOR HER.

- The birth partner needs to ensure the mother is calm and relaxed. LEARN BREATHING OR CALMING MASSAGE TECHNIQUES.

STILL NEED CONVINCING?

- If it is still unclear why the Birth Partner has this important role to fulfil then I invite them to think of a time when they may have felt intimidated, threatened or fearful. Even if this situation hasn't occurred - how would their mind and body respond?

- Think about what you could do to help your partner feel safe.

- Keep the mother's zone "safe", make sure she knows you are there, present and connected to what she is doing. Labour is not a time for checking your mobile phone!

- This is a time when ALL of your focus should be on her. You may feel you're not doing much but _don't underestimate the reassurance your presence will have on her feeling protected and supported and loved._

- *The love hormone oxytocin and endorphins will help labour to flow and help with the natural cocktail of pain relief. The birth partner role is very important! :)*

PREPARATION

If you are tense or nervous your partner will pick up on this, this can slow down their labour as they may sense they are not being protected or they may feel they need to nurture / protect you. If this happens they will come out of their zone and the primitive part of the brain. It will impact the flow of labour in some way.

It is so essential that a birth partner understands the needs of a woman in labour, that they remain calm and relaxed and present throughout.

It is also essential that a birth partner prepares for the birth *with* the mother. Remember this is team work.

HOW YOU CAN DO THIS

Practicing relaxation together. I will share tips, relaxation scripts and resources that will help you both relax, it is important you both practice relaxation and breathing techniques.

Begin working on non-verbal communication with each other. In order to read a situation without a mother having to come out of her headspace the birth partner must be able to anticipate and understand the mothers needs.

A great way to practice this is through light touch massage during pregnancy. Initially communicating what the mothers preferences are in terms of strokes and pressure etc will be verbal however this will evolve so that the birth partner is more in tune with subtle changes in response.

Light touch massage is also a great way during pregnancy to stimulate the beautiful hormones required to help labour flow and act as a natural form of pain relief

Gentle words and encouragement during birth can also
work well to encourage a birthing woman. (This will be
covered more in a later section.)

Questions to consider for your birth preferences:

How does your partner feel about pain relief such as an epidural?
What pain relief feels acceptable to your partner? (This may change
on the day if contractions are strong, your partner is tired or feels
pressurised, or if your partner is induced)

Birth can deviate from a 'plan' and this is to be expected so just have
an idea of what you would both like and inform yourself about the
options the pros and cons and what your values are.

What is your combined view of what is deemed as risk and what
questions would you ask on your partners behalf?

Other things to consider are optimal cord clamping, Vitamin K
injection, Syntocin, skin to skin contact, breast feeding or bottle
feeding.

There are many more options you may want to be clear on and this
list is not conclusive...

Together you should also start to discuss birth preferences. Here is something to get you started;

RECAP

In this section you have learnt:

- How the primitive part of our brain is used for birth
- Why the birth environment needs to feel safe for a birthing woman
- Sphincters Law and what is needed to enable the opening of a woman's cervix
- One role of the birthing partner to "protect" the mother and her environment

EXERCISE:

- Moo! Next time you poo!
- Begin preparing for the birth together
- Try some of the other sounds together
- Think about how as a birth partner you can begin to establish regular non verbal communication if you don't already.

To begin with you may need to communicate and ask what the mother needs from you right now. As you become more in tune and your bond strengthens you can ease labour and aid in the flow....this ties in with the powerful love hormone oxytocin - up next!

7.
OXYTOCIN

Oxytocin is the love hormone responsible for helping induce a restful, calm, state. For women in a pre and postnatal state is Oxytocin is responsible for managing pain in childbirth, helping birth to flow naturally due to the relaxed physiological state. The flow of oxytocin ties in with non verbal communication and what your partner can do to help you and enable this wonderful hormone to be present.

Here are a few ideas to consider to help the oxytocin flow. Think about what your partner likes?

- Candles
- A romantic meal
- Walks along the beach or in the woods
- Massages, hand massages, back and shoulder massages
- Certain music
- A soak in the bath, prepared by you.
- Looking at special photographs of family, friends, a holiday, wedding

- You doing something she always does and letting her do something for herself instead
- Slow dancing in the kitchen
- Watching comedy or cheesy romantic comedies (I know but this is all about her feeling good!)
- Foot rub
- Playing with her hair
- Massaging her tummy (and connecting with your baby!)
- Talking to your baby, reading to your baby or playing him or her music
- Telling her why you love her
- Tell her how beautiful she looks, how incredible her body is as this tiny human grows

<u>Do what you know she will like and if you're not sure then ask her.</u>

I had one woman say that she loved her husband reading to her. If that works then do it!

Personally in the early stages of my second labour when we were slowly waiting and easing into the birth experience we played Scrabble! I'm a Scrabble geek and I love it. What can I say? It made me happy and relaxed and I breathed through those early contractions whilst still playing and I won.

So what makes your partners oxytocin flow?

8.
PAIN RELIEF

NATURAL PAIN RELIEF OPTIONS

WATER

Whether it's a shower running down your back, a bath, birthing pool. Water soothes and relaxes the mind and the body, turning down the dial on the intensity of the contractions. Be mindful a bath is great in the early stages of active labour yet water creates buoyancy which goes against gravity. A soothing shower may be great if your feel you would rather stand AND get the benefit of gravity

If you immerse yourself in a birthing pool too soon this could slow down labour, so the second stage of labour is preferable. (Process of labour is covered later in this guide.)

CHANGING POSITION

This may seem surprising however, by attending a good pregnancy yoga class or similar you will learn different positions and how they will be beneficial for birth. Familiarisation will mean that during labour they are instinctual. For example being on all fours may offer your back some relief. Using a birthing ball may also help your back whilst still making use of gravity. Standing and leaning against a wall rotating or swaying your hips will relax you and help calm your mind. So think about, or rather practice various positions so movement can provide relief.

NATUROPATHY/ HOMEOPATHY

More people are using old wisdom when it comes to health and well-being, there are many options in terms of diet, nutrition that can be beneficial prior to birth such as consuming dates weeks before has been proven to help prepare the cervix for birth, raspberry leaf tea prior to birth is also beneficial. Kiwi fruits for after birth to help you after birth to go to the toilet. The softer your stool the better.

I also used a Childbirth Homeopathic kit, you can buy these cheaply and the contents can be used in the future for other health needs too. This can be particularly helpful should fears arise, the homeopathy will support you through the phases of labour depending on your circumstances. Each kit comes with a guide of how to use it.

REFLEXOLOGY

Regular reflexology during pregnancy can help in so many ways, I'm not an expert however it is said to help with hormone balance, posture and alignment, some people use reflexology to encourage their baby to turn if they are laying in a breach position. A bit like posture and alignment practice in yoga, reflexology will also contribute to helping birth flow more easily. Preparation as always for birth is key.

HEAT PACK

Some people find that a heat pack on their sacrum is beneficial to ease the sensation of the contractions across their back.

TENS

This is a device that creates electrical impulses on either side of your spine. Effectiveness can vary, it may help some people more than others. If your baby is back to back then a lot of these women will find it provides more relief.

ACCUPUNCTURE/ ACCUPRESSURE

Similar to reflexology this is another way in which we can prepare our body for birth. We naturally produce the hormones and endorphins needed to enable birth to flow naturally.

MASSAGE

In labour, massage is important because it brings you close to the person who is caring for you. The touch of someone who loves you and wants to help you is very empowering when you're coping with contractions and are perhaps tired and frightened.

Very importantly, massage can inhibit the release of adrenaline, which can hinder the progress of labour.

Stimulating the skin also helps release oxytocin, it will expel the placenta after birth and promote feelings of attachment and bonding between mother and baby.

The priority as always is to ensure that the mother is feeling safe, supported and cared for.

9.
INTERVENTION & B.R.A.I.N

BE PREPARED FOR THE UNEXPECTED

When the natural flow of labour is prohibited in some way medical interventions are often offered or sometimes it is deemed necessary by a health professional to advise that an intervention is required that you hadn't expected. Be sure always to ask questions if you can and understand the implications of the recommended actions.

For example if you have one intervention it could lead to others as your natural flow is being interrupted or sped up. A medical pain relief option could slow labour down or have other adverse affects. Often one intervention can lead to another intervention further along in the process, it can take labour off course like a domino effect. Be mindful of this and make a decision with this knowledge in mind, having assessed yourselves your options and what you think is best for you. Take on board medical advice and also trust your instincts and your body, sometimes as a labouring mother you know what you need however we doubt ourselves.

Start practicing the use of the BRAIN Acronym now in everyday life

When making any decisions in labour use your BRAIN.

B - What are the BENEFITS of this course of action?

R - What are the RISKS?

A - Are there any ALTERNATIVES?

I - What are the IMPLICATIONS of following this course of action? Will it make further INTERVENTIONS more likely?

N - What if we do NOTHING and wait an hour or two before doing anything?

Discuss your birth preferences and make sure you are both aware of what you would like to happen in birth.

You need to ensure you are on the same page, however if your pregnant partner changes her mind, listen and talk about it. Sometimes this can be an <u>instinctive</u> preference and choice. Be patient.

As a birthing partner you need to show solidarity during pregnancy, keep the vibe and energy positive as this will carry through to the birth.

Preparing for the birth together by doing things like reading this guide, making time to both practice relaxation techniques together whether that's through an MP3, relaxation scripts, breathing or massage are all a great way to build on the non verbal communication.

The time you invest communicating now and understanding non verbal queues, understanding where your partners mind is at..... ALL of this will help you support your partner in birth. She will need to feel understood without having to speak, she will need to feel safe, protected, loved and supported by you. This will undoubtedly help the experience be more positive for both of you.

RECAP

- A positive mindset can really help you move forward in a way that is best for you no matter what turns the birth experience may take.

- Look at what will make you both feel more positive about birth and what fears you need to let go of.

- Immerse yourself in positive birth stories.

- Practice relaxations together scripts / audio.

- Work out what affirmations work for you now and will in labour.

- Create a vision board or work out what visual aids may help oxytocin and confidence flow.

- Communication about what helps your partner feel relaxed / feel good.

- Practice breathing techniques.

- Sphincters law - Moo when you poo ;-)

10.
RELAXATION IN PREGNANCY

Pregnancy can be an exciting and nervous time. Relaxation is often undervalued however it is vital as the baby needs as much as it can get from the mother, which can leave the mother exhausted and emotional. If suffering from morning sickness, headaches and lack of sleep then relaxation can help to combat this.

Time to relax and focus on you and nurturing yourself and your unborn baby can also give you an opportunity to bond with your baby. It's a double win.

It's important to keep stress levels as low as possible in pregnancy as studies have shown that the stress hormone, cortisol can reach the baby. This isn't shared here to cause more undue stress or any guilt, we all have stressors in life and this can not always be avoided. Yet, it is important to remember that if mum is relatively relaxed throughout pregnancy then instead of cortisol, endorphins and oxytocin will be released and both of these help people feel good! This is fantastic for the mother's well being and the baby will receive these feel good hormones too.

Why is *practicing* relaxation important?

There are so many more reasons that relaxation is important. Relaxation can help a woman prepare mentally and emotionally throughout pregnancy for the labour ahead and the arrival of their baby. To be able to easily relax the body and mind in challenging or fraught moments in the babies early weeks will be invaluable, enabling the mother to tune into her instincts rather than be in a heightened state of stress when it is more difficult to make decisions.

Relaxation is restorative, even a few minutes of relaxing breathing techniques, or body scan to soften the whole body can work wonders on our emotional and physical state.

During pregnancy our immune system is low and therefore if we can practice relaxation we can be less susceptible to prolonged bouts of illness.

Relaxation can also help with sleeplessness and anxiety, some mothers suffer with insomnia with the impending birth of their baby and so a well practiced body scan relaxation can ease you into a restful , restorative sleep..

Relaxation can help deal with pregnancy ailments and discomfort. If our minds are calm then any discomfort seems to lessen or at the very least the relaxed state can take the edge off whatever ailment we are dealing with.

Relaxation releases endorphins and oxytocin which help a woman to feel good and reaches the baby. What a great reason to book the massage or reflexology appointment! It's for both of you!

Relaxation gives a mother rest whilst her baby grow and at the same time as we learn to relax it can help us adjust to a new pace of life with a newborn. Perhaps a slower one than we may be used to in our everyday life.

Relaxation can help with exhaustion and feeling emotional because it restores and centres us. A time set aside for relaxation during the day can give us the energy boost we need for the rest of the day. This will be a great habit to adopt when the baby arrives because we need to make use of the opportunities that present themselves to relax to maintain the stamina required to take care of a new born.

Relaxation when pregnant can also help you bond and connect with your baby. This is special time to think about the baby you are growing inside, under your heart and in your womb. It can be time to pause and appreciate the blessing you have.

The more you can practice relaxation in pregnancy the more you can put it to use in labour, the more relaxed you are the more your body will be able to do what it is designed to do without your mind and body being tense and making the process more challenging. Tension will work against you, relaxation will work for you. Essential in labour!

So, practice practice practice.

What can you do to relax and nurture your unborn baby?

- MP3s /Audios of relaxation tracks
- Pregnancy massage
- Pregnancy yoga
- Relaxing bath
- Reflexology
- Reiki
- Meditation
- Visualisation
- Music
- Manicure/Pedicure :-)
- Cup of tea (with no distractions!)
- Going for a walk
- Enjoying nature
- Mindfully be in the present
- Sleep/Rest
- Aromatherapy

BIRTH PARTNER - Understanding how your partner relaxes and perhaps try to read scripts provided in this guide to her, know what will help her and find out now, practice together e.g. use of certain word or phrases, understanding which breathing technique works for your partner, understanding what kind of environment your partner needs in order to feel safe and secure to birth. This is essential homework.

Why is relaxation in childbirth important?

As mentioned fear or tension in labouring women can inhibit the natural progress of labour, however, positive hormones will help labour and allow it to progress naturally. Oxytocin and endorphins are opiate-like hormones and reduce the feelings of pain, therefore the more relaxed a mother in labour is the better able to manage the pain of contractions. The more relaxed the mother is the more intuitively she is able to follow her body's needs and the more easily the muscles of the uterus and cervix will open and thin. We know that a relaxed jaw is proven to help open a woman's cervix so if a woman is relaxed she can gently allow her body to do what it needs to do without her body tensing and holding back.

It is important that a mother feels safe and secure in her environment so anything else that can be done to help make her feel calm and relaxed should be considered.

- Breathing techniques can help calm the mind, as can some movements learnt in pregnancy yoga classes
- Dim lights
- Music
- Candles
- Aromatherapy
- Light touch massage
- Who is present at the birth supporting you
- The right kind of verbal or non verbal encouragement and support

Relaxation in birth comes with feeling positive, calm, trusting our body's innate wisdom to give birth, feeling protected (with the help of the environment and a birthing partner) and feeling loved and supported throughout.

11.
BREATH

YOUR BREATH IS YOUR SUPER POWER

There are various breathing techniques you can use to help you during birth to remain calm, focused and help with pain relief. Regular practice is ideal beforehand to help you both on the day. When practicing breathing techniques and relaxation here are my top tips:

- Ensure you are relaxing your jaw and shoulders
- The longer the breath out as you exhale the further your baby is able to move down the birth canal
- Remember you can use Golden Thread breathing technique at any time not just during birth. It will calm your CNS and heart rate.
- Whenever your mind becomes busy bring your attention back to your breath.

Breathwork enables you to following your body's guidance rather than what is happening externally, it takes you inwards so that your body can do the work for you without your mind getting in the way.

By keeping your breath calm and steady through labour we allow the body, the abdominal muscles, your uterus to do what it is designed to do, contract so that it can push the baby down and out. The process is perfectly designed however we have learnt to fear it, so we tense and work against the body's natural instinct. Just like your body knows how to expel when you're on the toilet, the body knows how to birth a baby, even if your mind doesn't. So staying relaxed, practicing breathing techniques will help you surrender to what your body needs to do and you can work with it rather than against it.

When we are tense, under stress, fearful we tighten our pelvic floor, our pelvic tension is linked to how we are breathing. So slowing down our breath will tell our brain we are safe, which then aids the process letting the baby move down easier.

Contrary to what you may have seen on TV and films you are not constantly pushing, the way birth can be portrayed is far from the way in which we birth when connected to our bodies and our breath. The breath and how your baby moves is going to be different from one person to the next. Some people will birth their baby using involuntary pushing and their breath will be complimenting this, perhaps pausing in a reflexive way. In other cases when there is guided pushing then this may alter the pace of birth and if you are going against your natural instinct and this could cause a tear so follow what your body is telling you to do.

In terms of preparation if you don't already practice regular breath work then begin by noticing your breathing more, perhaps knowing that every time you inhale deeply you are sending vital nutrients to your unborn baby. It's such a good thing!

Practice breathing techniques whenever you feel slight tension or stress. I used to practice when in a queue at a supermarket, calm breath in long slow breath out. Someone asked me once if I was ok and I explained how I was practicing my breathing techniques. It's important not to feel self conscious about your breath, don't be afraid of it embrace the sound as you inhale and exhale. It's a sign you are alive!

Another great time to practice breathing techniques is when you have something causing discomfort, or as we have ailments in pregnancy such as aching hips or pelvis this is another good time to put your breath to good use and get endorphins flowing through your body.

A couple of suggestions for incorporating breath work;

VARIATIONS
- Use the Body Scan relaxation (in resources) to help
   you relax your entire body, it is perfect to practice

anytime, maybe in bed if your restless or on a
commute.
- Perhaps try to focus on breathing in calm/ love/
confidence and when you breath out release any
tension or fear
- You can also count IN 234 and OUT 2345... as close to
10 as possible.

The breath is probably the most important thing to practice. If you can use your breath in any situation to remain calm or to help you focus and go inwards then at any point it will anchor you and empower you.

So underrated but of such high importance, not just for pregnancy and birth but for life.

12.
VISUALISATION & AFFIRMATIONS

IF IT'S GOOD ENOUGH FOR WORLD CLASS ATHLETES......

Affirmations help prepare your mind and create new neural pathways in your brain and thought processes and affirmations work alongside knowing and understanding the capabilities of our bodies.

Affirmations such as these are powerful reminders that will support you. Practice them, say out loud those that resonate with you the most. Here are a few that are favourites and a list of more affirmations is provided in the resources. Pick and choose your favourites or tweak them to suit you better.

"My surges can not be bigger than me because they are me"
"I fully relax so my body can birth this baby"
"I relax my jaw"
"I trust my body and it's ability to birth"
" I am strong and capable"

" I open gently and with ease"

There is also a list of affirmations for the birth partner that they may like to use during labour to provide verbal confirmation and support. Ensure you run through these beforehand as it is important they work for her benefit.

Visualisations are also very powerful, they are used by a lot of successful people including world class athletes. The more you can run through something in your mind the more you can convince your brain this has already happened and your mind and body will respond in a similar way to how you've rehearsed.

You can start with something simple like imagining or visualising your baby in the ideal position, then you can visualise yourself opening up in labour and how calm you both are regardless of the environment, you can even visualise your baby descending efficiently, smoothly and gently into the world and you can imagine holding your baby close to you. Visualise the labour and how you would like it to go. Whilst it may not play out exactly as you'd like being in a mindset of a positive experience will help you to remain empowered during labour.

Think about other senses too, how can you feel calm, strong, in tune with your instincts and the sound of your breath? You may have music in the background you may use a pregnancy safe essential oil to help you focus your mind and connect you to your affirmations and visualisations.

I have recommended clients create a vision board, this is another way to help the visualisation process and pin point what words, images work for you and your oxytocin. You can incorporate visual images or affirmations that will help you feel calm. confident and empowered, use images that will help you remain focused the end goal and that will help your oxytocin to flow. Perhaps use your baby scan pictures picture, or a family image or a holiday picture with your partner. Perhaps have your babies first baby grow or outfit that brings back happy memories. Ensure it is somewhere yo ucan see it so at a glance when you need it the right image or affirmation is there reminding you of the outcome you want and how capable you are. If you plan to give birth in a hospital environment then I would suggest one you can fold up (made of card) so it can stand up on a table or chair - it needs to be where you can see it or touch it...

13.
PROCESS OF LABOUR

First Stage
The first stage of labour can start weeks, days or hours before the birth. When you begin to feel twinges or tightenings, pay attention, these may be Braxton Hicks and these are signs your body and your baby are preparing themselves for birth.

The first stage may begin by there being a "show", this is a mucus plug, sealing the cervix, which is expelled during the hours, sometimes days before labour. You may not even notice it.

Your waters MIGHT break, a sudden flood of water or a trickle, when this happens let the midwife know however there is no need to panic. Ensure the waters are CLEAR if not this could be a sign of meconium and you will likely be encouraged to go into hospital for monitoring.

When the time is getting closer usually the last few days of pregnancy, an amazing hormone called PROSTAGLANDIN is released. This hormone softens and thins the cervix, ripening you for birth! (TIP: Eating dates from 36 weeks, approximately 6 a day will help this process)

Contractions are phenomenal, imaging the muscles contracting to massage your baby out, the more you relax, as previously mentioned, the more easily your body can do what it is innately designed to do, i.e. feral ejection. So as your uterus is contracting and softening the cervix is opening to enable the baby to be born. Every contraction opens you up a little more. At this stage the female gets restless, she feels like moving around and these are our primitive instincts helping baby to get into position.

A natural cocktail of pain relieving hormones are released at this time, oxytocin and endorphins, this is the time to trust your body and work with it, relax and breathe.

Your body does it all. Trust it. Yield to it. Work with it.

Contractions are about 15 minutes apart however can be longer. It's a gradual build-up and the contractions gradually become closer together and more powerful.

Use your breath to get you through every contraction and remember *every out breath brings you one step closer to meeting your baby.* Golden thread breathing technique is perfect for this stage. Conserve as much energy as possible before the second stage of labour.

Try to stay at home for as long as you can, make it beautiful birth preparation space and savour the experience of intimate, quiet time for just the two of you for as long as you can.

Second Stage

Once the cervix is completely open, the body really mobilises itself to help your baby be born Earth side.

The mother may go into her own deeper primal zone, if she isn't there already. She may make sounds you've never heard before. She may not want to speak. She may not want to listen. She may not want to be touched. This stage is the transition when fear and doubt kick in. This is natures deliberate way of letting your adrenalin kick in. This stage means your baby is nearly here and it's the final stage using your final reserves of energy to bring your baby into the world.

Contractions become stronger and more intense because they have to contract the uterus even more to push/ breathe the baby out. Your baby is very nearly here!

Keep using gravity and breath and right at the end there is another big rush of oxytocin as your baby is born. This design helps a mother to bond with her baby, however depending on the labour and external factors or perhaps due to exhaustion, the mother may not have the rush of oxytocin and that is perfectly ok. Some women feel a rush of love immediately after birth, however this is rarer than people realise. This is no reflection on the mother and can be for many reasons, the type of birth, intensity of the birth, shock. It can take time to fall in love with your baby as you get to know them and that's ok.

Third Stage

Oxytocin and endorphins should flood you. Contractions continue and you will then birth the placenta.

Note: You may want /need an injection to help the placenta to detach from the uterus wall. Sometimes the midwifes will massage your tummy for the placenta to come out, be prepared for losing blood. Be sure to research whether you want the injection and all research at what point you would like the umbilical cord cut. There are studies that show leaving the umbilical cord attached will benefit the baby as they will receive all kinds of goodness, nutrients, stem cells etc from the placenta even after both are birthed.

14.
IMPORTANCE OF AN ACTIVE BIRTH

"I LIKE TO MOVE IT MOVE IT!"

WHY AN ACTIVE BIRTH?

Rumour has it that the reason women have been lying on our backs to give birth for hundreds of years is because of Louis XIV. What he knew about childbirth is anyone's guess however he apparently wanted to watch the birth of his son. He insisted he watch from the end of the bed whilst his baby was being born which meant his lucky lady had to lie on her back so he could get a good view!

Then what follows is a new fashion or trend which involves a women laying on a bed to birth, far more "upmarket" than squatting and being on all fours which although more practical was animalistic and "common"!

It was also deemed much easier for the obstetrician to monitor, heaven forbid we make it hard for the person observing than the mother bringing a new life into the world!

It makes much more sense logically that for anything to come out we use gravity to help us, lying on our back is not making use of gravity! Also this is narrowing our pelvis and making it harder for our baby to turn.

Think about taking a ring off your finger that's a bit tight do you just leave your finger straight and pull it over your knuckle or do you have to move it, wriggle it a little, bend your finger perhaps? Movement is important for helping your baby move through the pelvis.

The best way to know how to move when you can't see what is going on is to move how your body and instincts are telling you. Step into that "animalistic" primitive part of your brain, relax and simply listen, if a voice in your head say's "I need to squat" then squat! If it say's " go on all fours" then go on all fours.

Just stay off your back! Being immobile will work against you and your baby.

Tune in to what feels comfortable for you. Tune into the communication from your baby, this is completely possible the more relaxed you are and in a calm, safe and supportive environment.

Listen to your body, with every movement and posture. Learn to let go, surrender, all you need to do is listen to your body and your baby. Move as you feel you need to move, squat, stand, all fours whatever works for you.

Surrender, let go, you do not need to do anything except relax, breath, listen and move.

15.
BIRTHING POSITIONS

YOUR BIRTH PARTNER IS YOUR PILLAR OF STRENGTH

If we want to make use of gravity, movement, open poses, the security of having our partners near, oxytocin and endorphins then couples birthing positions can really help. Benefits are also maximum circulation between mother and baby, better alignment of the baby to pass through the pelvis, stronger rushes, Increased pelvic diameters when squatting or kneeling AND active involvement and support from your partner!

Here are a few positions that you can do together, the birthing partner, the intimacy, support will all assist in a positive birth experience.

The Slow Dance
Arms can be round the back of your birth partners neck, or they could be round your partners waist. Slow dance, or just sway rhythmically. Or let yourself hang. Listen to your partners heart beat or look into their eyes, enjoy the closeness whilst being supported and conserving energy.

RECOMMENDED - If you want to use a standing position for a while then your partners should ideally be leaning with their back against a wall. Your partner will need support too whilst supporting you in labour. They could be there a while just like you.

Forehead Rest
With your birthing partners back against the wall, rest your forehead or head in a way that's comfortable for you against their chest or on their shoulder. Sway from side to side with your legs apart for balance. This can help you shut out what is going on around you and get into your mental 'zone'.

Facing Grip and Semi Squat
With your birthing partners back against the wall their elbows at their side and lower arms forward with palms facing up or perhaps with clenched fists. The birthing mother holds on to the lower arms with her hands just below her partners elbows. Either stand like this moving in a way that feels comfortable or you could widen your stance and squat if this feels right for you. If you squat then your partner will hold on to your arms too. Squatting can also work with both of you facing away from the wall being supported by her arms over the top of her partners extended lower arms.

RECOMMENDED - With positions kneeling on the floor you may want cushions under your knees. Also think about the angle of your back, the more upright you are in these poses the better use of gravity.

Sit with Child
The birth partner can be sitting in a chair with their partner kneeling in front of them on the floor, resting her arms on their partners legs or resting them around the back of his neck.

Sit and be open
As with Sit and Child above however with one leg up, foot on the floor creating an open pelvis.

Sit and Squat
As above but squatting facing her birth partner or away from her birth partner.

Yoga Ball Massage
The birthing mother can be on a yoga ball receiving light touch massage with her partner sitting behind her in a chair.

Yoga Ball
Circles and rocking whilst sitting on the ball are great to help dilation. Keep your upper back straight so you're just using your lower spine and pelvis to move your baby.

16.
LIGHT TOUCH MASSAGE

Light touch massage is a great way to release endorphins and encourage oxytocin. It is a form of pain relief so often overlooked.

To get started find a comfortable position for both of you. Tell your birth partner where it hurts or aches and when they begin to massage they should lean as opposed to use their strength to apply pressure when it's needed. Pressure on areas like the sacrum really can provide great relief during pregnancy and during labour.

As with everything in this guide, practice these during pregnancy, this will help with the non verbal communication which will be hugely beneficial during birth and it is also a great opportunity for the birth partner to bond with the baby before it is born.

Here are a few options to get you started;

MASSAGE BETWEEN CONTRACTIONS

Simple light and relaxing fingertip strokes down either side of the spine or a relaxing foot massage.
The aim is to encourage relaxation and let the woman recover.

Spinal Strokes

Start at the nape of the neck and sweep down to the base of the spine. Using alternate hands work either side of the spine NOT on it. Keep continuous movement by using one hand after another, always leaving one hand in contact.

Massage During Contractions

Generally, massage around the sacral area and on the lower back, buttocks and thighs is most effective. The strokes should be deep and done smoothly and rhythmically. Abdominal massage can be useful but use very gentle strokes.

In all cases be guided as to whether the woman wants it. Don't be disappointed if your partner doesn't want a massage. It's not uncommon for some women not to want to be touched during the second stage of labour.

Sacral Circles

Find the flat bone at the bottom of the spine. This is the sacrum. Use one hand to support the front of the hipbone. Use the heel of the other hand to apply some pressure on the sacrum (remember to check the pressure with your partner) and keeping the pressure even, slowly move round in small circles.

Sacral Snake

Using the heel of the hand move from the far left to right. Return to the left using the hand in a wriggly movement.

Sacral Heart

Using the flats of both the hands start at the base of the spine. Push up when the woman breathes out, making a heart shape back to starting position on breathing in.

Sacral Warmth

Push gently on the sacrum to warm the area. Repeat as many times and at a pace that is comfortable for your partner.

SUPPORTED POSITIONS FOR MASSAGE

These techniques may be beneficial during the second stage as you will need to be upright in a forward leaning position.

Lean forward onto a pillow, yoga ball or beanbag. Spread your knees wide. If you are massaging, always remember to check now and then if your partner still wants to be massaged.

DURING CONTRACTIONS

Buttock Kneading
Knead your partner's buttocks with the flat part of both fists. Turn the fist outwards during the contraction to intensify pressure.

Hip Massage
Put the heels of your hands centrally at the base of the spine. Lean forward and push outwards across buttocks to hips. Glide hands back to starting position as your partner breathes in.

BETWEEN CONTRACTIONS

Sweeping Strokes
Start at the base of the spine. Move both hands smoothly up either side of the spine up to the neck. Move the hands round the shoulders and glide back down to the base of the spine.

Foot Massage
If you are sitting on a stool or are in a reclining position, then a lovely foot massage between contractions can also help greatly with relaxation.

17
HOW IT ALL COMES TOGETHER

We have covered many different aspects of birth preparation in this guide, so how does it all come together?

Think of this like a checklist, if all factors are known and you are able to prepare then you are in a a much better position to have an empowered positive birth. Everything in this guide mentioned are big contributing factors to a flowing physiological birth.

To set the scene;

You are both relaxed and calm in an environment that is nurturing and helps your oxytocin flow. Perhaps the lights are dim and you have fairy lights or candles lit, feel good music playing, whatever is right for you. You understand what is happening to your body in the first stages of labour and you are happy sitting on a yoga ball enjoying the moment, in your zone with your breath. When a contraction happens you know you need to relax more fully and your breath helps you go more inward. Perhaps you get up and move to lean on a wall and circle your hips or perhaps your body is telling you to squat so you squat. You are instinctively doing what YOU need.

You have already dealt with any fears that you may have had and you have researched the possible options you may be offered, you already know the benefits and potential implications of various courses of action and intervention and between you and your birth partner you are on the same page. You have been practicing the use of the B.R.A.I.N. acronym and so can make informed rational decisions based on what is right for you.

Your birth partner can communicate for you if needed to keep you in your 'zone'. Your birth partners presence is reassuring and their strength and support is exactly what you need, perhaps affirmations and encouragement when needed or laughter and a slow dance to keep the love hormones flowing. Light touch massage, drinks and snacks to keep you hydrated. You are being take care of so you can take care of the important role of bringing your baby Earth side.

You are able to relax when you need to, using the relaxation scripts either by listening to them or by knowing them in your mind and associating them with a calm breathing technique that works for you. Perhaps having paired your relaxation practice with a relaxing essential oil blend you can more easily physically relax when you smell the blend.

You are so in tune and relaxed that although contractions may be strong you do not fear them as you know they are only temporary and you understand that your body is doing something it is perfectly designed to do. You trust your instincts so if something doesn't seem right you will be vocal and confident in expressing any concerns.

You move through the processes of labour and understand that at some point you may have doubts about your abilities and this may be the transition from first to second stage, whereby your adrenalin may help you to birth your baby. This is all perfectly designed, perhaps you use homeopathy to help you at this time. You continue to move instinctively into positions that work for you, even if it means it is not how you visualised your birth you trust the process.

Your birth partner is a constant source of strength and encouragement, even if that is by remaining quietly by your side. Together you ensure you can handle any surprises that come your way, your birth goes smoothly and your baby has the best start possible.

This is how your babies life begins and how the journey into parenthood begins.

THIS is how everything you learn can come together. Invest in this positive experience with time and team work.

18
THE FOURTH TRIMESTER

"THE FORGOTTEN TRIMESTER"

THE FOURTH TRIMESTER

This is the first three months after your baby has been born and is new to the world. This period of time is an important time to help your baby adjust to being in the world and an important time for bonding to occur between mother and baby. It is also a crucial time for a new mother to heal her body, rest and restore her energy.

In some cultures a mother is allowed to 'retreat' from the outside world when her baby is born. Someone will come and take care of her, ensure she eats well and has time to physically heal and bond with her baby.

Chinese tradition of care postnatally is called zuo yuezi and is focussed on nourishing a new mother and helping them to thrive after birth. They believe that during the Fourth Trimester, the first three months post birth, the healing time will help a mother preserve her reproductive health for future children or eventually experience an easier menopause.

The Physical
You will bleed for some weeks after birth, this varies on the type of birth and allowing yourself to heal. If you invest in placenta encapsulation bleeding usually stops within a couple of weeks, without and it may be longer.

You are healing after growing a baby for the best part of a year! Your baby has used all the goodness you have in order to grow and thrive. Now is time for you to restore your body, allow it to heal itself. You may feel great and this is the hormones, adrenalin and excitement. STILL you need to take it easy!

You have also given birth and regardless of the type of birth, you need to heal. Imagine running a marathon without resting after and continuing as normal in the fast past world we live in and with a new baby!

You still have the hormone relaxin in your body which helped your body to prepare for baby's growth and birth, this means you're still vulnerable to injury lifting and doing heavy lifting, moving etc. You may find after birth your feet and legs sometimes ache and click. This is relatively normal as your body is settling back now your baby is earth side.

Paternity leave is often over in a couple of weeks and a mother is then left to deal with a new baby and look after her own health and wellbeing. The irony is that for the first couple of weeks babies mostly sleep, this is so that the mother can rest and recuperate after bringing her baby into the world. Birth partners should be nurturing the mother as much as possible in the fourth trimester. After only a couple of weeks your baby will become more "lively" and demanding yet this is often when a mum is without her partner. We need to be very mindful of this.

Relationships will evolve too as you undoubtedly have less time for each other. Sometimes partners can feel pushed away and they can also lack confidence with their baby when they return to work as it's often the mother that is at home learning the baby's cues.

It is commonly underestimated how long it will take a woman to recover from creating a life and bringing that life into the world, regardless of the birth experience. It takes a full year for a woman to physically recover and the fourth trimester is the foundation of that healing. It's vital to take things slowly and do as little as possible. In addition to the healing that is taking place there may also be feelings of isolation, feelings of overwhelm, exhaustion and hormones to deal with. This period of adjustment for the mother and baby is incredibly important to be sensitive about.

The emotional and hormonal
Depending on your birth experience and your pregnancy you may be high on oxytocin and adrenalin for a while.

Baby blues is only a period of a couple of days soon after birth. If you are suffering with low mood for longer than a couple of days talk to your midwife, health visitor or GP. Postnatal depression impacts 1 in 4 women and doesn't discriminate. Seek help or advice and don't suffer unduly. Note: Fathers can also experience post natal depression.

Your life has changed. Well it doesn't take a rocket scientist to figure this one out BUT often new parents can feel overwhelmed with the responsibility. I have heard so often "I didn't realise it would be as hard as this", in honesty ALL mothers and parents feel like this.

You're adjusting to life as a new mum/parent, the learning curve is steep! We will make mistakes and we must forgive ourselves quickly. Make sure that you ask for help when you need it, you need to make sure you are ok. If you are then you can better look after your baby and your family.

RECOMMENDATIONS

- Prepare healthy meals before your baby arrives that you can freeze or arrange for a friend, family member, neighbour to bring you fresh meals (without expecting an invite in - Unless of course it's to help with housework!)
- Keep visitors to a minimum, your baby has been in a tiny, safe, quiet space and is now exposed to so much more. Smell, louder noise, the feel of clothing and blankets, sun, wind, a new home which must feel HUGE to them. It's no wonder they want to be cuddled and feel safe in your arms.
- Do not try and do too much. Just rest as long as possible, now is a great time for cuddles and watching a great series on TV from the comfort of your sofa
- You should be focussed on your recovery and bonding with your baby as much as you can, particularly if there are older siblings, the new dynamic that a baby brings, it's an adjustment for everyone, take it slow and steady.
- If you can get a sling then this will be great for you and your baby. You'll feel you can do a little more with your hands free and you baby will be close to you still. There are loads of benefits to sling wearing, check out the local sling libraries before your baby arrives so you know where to go.

- Isolation can be hard as a new mum, whilst it's important not to do too much, try to speak to people or meet people for a cuppa when you feel up to it.
- Sometimes just going for a brief walk each day can make you feel physically and mentally refreshed.
- Please do not try to lose weight too soon. You're body is amazing and has done something incredible! It takes a year for your body to recover from pregnancy and birth and even then you may find your body shape has changed. This is normal and actually your new softness is great for your baby, comforting and reassuring.
- Enjoy your baby and if there are any struggles know that you aren't alone, there are mothers around the world going through the same as you.

19.
CONCLUSION

BIRTH PARTNER RECAP

- Make sure your partner feels safe and secure in her environment and with the people around her
- Practice light touch massage but don't be offended if she doesn't want to be touched
- Try to create an environment suitable for birth, scents, LED candles or real candles if at home, dim lights, music to help her relax.
- Protect her space when she needs it
- Be near even if she does not want to speak or be touched
- Maintain ownership of your birth experience, these are your choices, consent is important
- Know that our bodies are amazing, a woman can grow life without interventions so should trust our body to give birth
- Remember an active birth using gravity is best and will help your partner and your baby
- Remain calm yourself
- You may want to protect your partner and be concerned, the best way to help your partner is to be calm and let her know you are physically there, you

are in this together, your mere presence is valuable and supportive even if you feel you aren't doing anything.

20.
RESOURCES

RELAXATION SCRIPT 1 (Golden Thread)
To be read slowly by the birth partner or recorded one of
you to listen to regularly;

"Make sure you're comfortable and warm
Imagine a golden light shining on top of your head,
notice how your forehead feels, if you feel any tension
gently soften the brow.
Notice how your temples feel, cheeks and jaw,
If you notice tension in your jaw gently part your lips.

Notice how your neck and shoulders feel.
Allow the shoulders to drop.
Let the sensation of any tension travel down the arms
the elbows wrists and fingers.
Simply allow yourself to let go.
Notice now how your spine feels, notice if there is any
tension in your back or your hips.
Imagine that golden light travelling down the spine.
Don't change anything, just notice.

Now bring your awareness to your chest area notice if it feels tight.
Notice your breathing, are your breaths short and shallow or long and deep, again don't change anything.

Notice now how your mind is, is it active and busy struggling to settle? Or is it calm and focused, don't judge yourself or try to resist, it's natural for thoughts to come and go, when a thought comes welcome it, then imagine it like a fluffy white cloud and see it disappearing into the distance.
Bring your attention back to your breath, this helps to anchor the mind.
Now notice how you feel, notice if you are feeling happy sad, anxious or worried, again don't judge yourself, its normal for our moods to change as we deal with the ups and downs that life brings us.

Now bring your awareness to the tummy, (this can be where we hold the most tension), bring your hands to the belly and take a moment to visualise you're beautiful baby.
Be aware of this wonderful new life that you have created.
Notice if he or she is resting or busy, don't worry just know that you and your baby are safe and being taken care of by nature and the universe.
Feel that magical bond with your baby, you can gently rub your belly knowing this is a powerful way of communicating with your baby.

Inhale calm and peace, exhale tension or worries.

Now bring your awareness to the breath, you can keep your hands on the belly if you wish.
Take a full deep breath in expanding the belly and then through softly parted lips slowly breath out, making that exhalation last as long as you can.
Focus on breathing in love and positivity for yourself and as you breathe out any tension, negativity or anxiety you relax more deeply.
Just keep on breathing, in this way for a few breaths allowing yourselves to let go a little bit more with every breath.

If you want to you can count in 2, 3, 4, Out 2,3,4,5, as close to 10 as feels comfortable.

Or visualise a fine golden thread, with every slow breath out visualise gently blowing away further into the distance a beautiful fine golden thread.
With each breath the golden thread gently drifts further and further into the distance,
Each breath bringing you one step closer to meeting your beautiful baby"

RELAXATION SCRIPT 2

1. "All you need to do is to lie on your left hand side.
    Place a cushion under your belly and between your
    knees. Make sure you are comfortable and place a
    blanket over you.

2. Now close your eyes and listen to my voice.

3. Relaxation is a vital time to nurture you and your
    baby.

4. Imagine a beautiful golden light, is shining down on
    you and your baby. You are both safe.

5. Keep your breathing slow and rhythmic, knowing
    that with each breath you are cocooning your baby
    in beautiful calming vapour of silk.

6. Bring your awareness to your forehead, your
    temples and the crown of your head. Notice how it
    feels. If there is any tension, allow it to release.
    Soften your forehead and your temples. Allow your
    cheeks to release. Pay attention to your jaw. Allow it
    to drop and softly part your lips.

7. Move your awareness down to your neck and
    shoulders. Keep your neck and shoulders soft and
    just allow them to become heavy. Let all tension float
    away. Keep your breathing soft, gentle and slow.

8. Let your spine release. Know that the earth is supporting you and your baby and keeping you safe.

9. Allow your hips to spread and release. There is no effort required. Just allow yourself to let go.

10. Your legs, knees, feet and ankles are soft and heavy.

11. Now just allow yourself to lie in this position.

12. When you are ready to wake up, open your eyes gently and sit up very slowly. Take some deep breaths and allow yourself some time before standing up."

LIST OF BIRTH AFFIRMATIONS

She believed she could so she did
Soften, Open, Release
Each wave has a purpose
I am bringing my baby earth side
Birth is amazing no matter how it happens
My body is natural strong & perfect
I am focused on my calm gentle birth
I have faith in my body and its ability to birth my baby
I am a strong capable woman - Hear me roar!
I am built for birth, I've got this
Each contraction brings me one step closer to meeting
my baby
Relaxed jaw = soft cervix
I can do this
I was born to do this
My baby is in the perfect position for birth
My baby will birth easily because I am so relaxed
Birth is normal and natural
I am in complete control of my body and mind
I feel confident and safe
My job is to relax and allow birth to happen
I feel the love others have for me during the birth
I set aside my worries and allow my body to do its job
My surges can not be greater than me because they are
me
My body opens, my mind quiets, my baby descends
I trust my baby knows what to do
My baby and I work together

Each wave brings my baby closer to me
The knowledge to birth is deep within me
My pelvis is opening and releasing as have countless
women before me
Soft jaw, soft hands, slow breath
Open
Trust - Roar - Surrender - Relax - Breathe
My body will progress at its own pace, my body knows
what to do
My baby is the perfect size for my body
I birth with ease
Calmly I trust in my body to birth my baby
This will not last forever
Relax, Breath, Open
I soften, I open, I release
My body knows how to have this baby just as my body
knew how to grow this baby
I listen to my body
Move with your instincts
My baby is working with me
I have everything it takes to birth my baby
I put all fear aside and welcome my baby with happiness
and joy
I am totally relaxed and at ease
I am prepared to meet whatever turn my birthing takes
My muscles work in harmony to make birthing easier
I feel confident, safe and secure
My mind is relaxed my body is relaxed

Affirmations for the birth partner to use and provide encouragement in labour

It would be a good idea to discuss before hand which ones appeal and which ones she will not find helpful. These can all be subjective so there may be some that just don't feel right for her. You want to be her voice of calm, her voice of encouragement to override any fear, tiredness and to keep the oxytocin and endorphins flowing

You are amazing
You are beautiful
I love you
I believe in you and your ability to birth
I am with you
You are strong
Our baby will be here soon
You are doing so well
You can do this
Listen to your body
Move with your instincts
Relax
I am here
You are safe
Gently and calmly focus on your breath, long slow out breaths

CONSIDERATIONS FOR YOUR BIRTHING BAG

FOR BIRTH
Maternity notes
Your music
Your aromatherapy e.g Clary Sage
Vision board
MP3s or relaxation scripts
Everything that you may need to get your oxytocin flowing
Placenta encapsulation kit
Cooling Spray or flannel
Lip balm
TENS Machine
Bendy straws
Camera

FOR MUM
Something to wear in labour, a bra, vest or a nighty
Loose fitting clean clothes for after, perhaps another nighty
Socks
Big oversized underwear - several pairs
Maternity Pads
Breast Pads
Arnica
Snacks
Toiletries including tooth brush

FOR BIRTH PARTNER
Clean t shirt
Snacks
Drinks
Money if you going to hospital (car park)

FOR BABY
Vests, grow, hats
Nappies
Pre made formula even if you plan to breast feed (be
prepared just in case)
Blanket
Muslins
Car Seat to bring them home!

PTSD & PND SUPPORT

As someone who experienced a very difficult first birth and eighteen months of Post Natal Depression (PND) it is important to me that as few people go through what I did. If after birth you feel that your birth experience was traumatic in any way then I urge you to seek help. I recommend the Rewind Technique for birth which I have used on women over the years successfully. It will realign you and help you detach from the emotional turmoil the experience caused and help you move forward positively.

There are of course other services such as Missing Pieces which is an opportunity to go through your birth experience with a midwife who can help you understand what happened. This is sometimes all someone needs to help them move forward.

I also recommend that people look into Placenta Encapsulation during pregnancy as this is said to help with hormone rebalancing and will therefore support you emotionally as you heal after pregnancy and birth. Placenta encapsulation also has lots of other benefits for healing and breast feeding.

Make sure that you connect with other parents, being a new mum can be isolating. It's like starting a new job yet there is no one to ask, no manual to read and you have this baby you are trying to get to know, understand and learn about. A support network is important.

There are organisations and charities that can help you with PND and Perinatal anxiety, it is brave and courageous to ask for help when you need it and in the long term it will be the best thing for your baby if you seek help and support you need. As the expression goes " You can't pour from an empty cup".

As a new mother in particular, be kind to yourself, let yourself go through the process of Matrescence, this is the process of *becoming* a mother. You are not who you were and you too are born anew when your baby enters the world. It can take time to adjust so honour what you are becoming.

ABOUT THE AUTHOR

Thank you for reading this book and for your support.

Finally self publishing this guide has reminded me of how far I have come and I want to share with women that we can overcome anything. An experience for me that was one of the most challenging of my life, birth, trauma, PND for eighteen months actually became something that became a gift. From something so difficult I decided that others should not have to go through what I did and so I jumped ship from my corporate career, retrained to specialise in Women's Health and Wellbeing and have been able to help hundreds of women. I believe I have planted seeds of empowerment, confidence and positive birth experiences which will continue to grow as more people learn what they are capable of.

I hope reading this will be another of those seeds planted.

With the best of intentions for your journey ahead.

Much love

Clare

Xx